Soil Nutrition Handbook

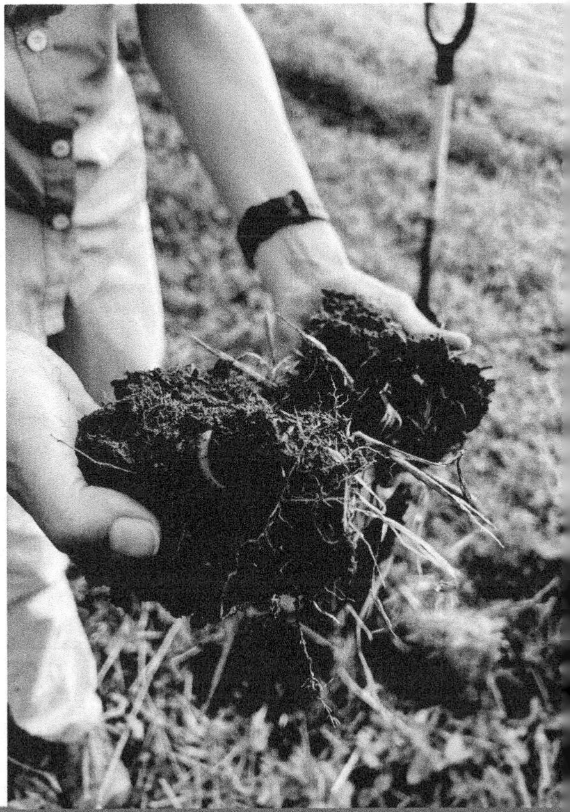

Understanding soil & soil reports

ACRES USA®
Published by Acres U.S.A.

By Mark Shepard and Gary Zimmer

About Acres U.S.A.

Founded in 1971 by Charles Walters, *Acres U.S.A.* magazine emerged from the need to promote ecological farming practices in a time when industrial agriculture was heavily reliant on synthetic fertilizers and pesticides. Inspired by figures like Rachel Carson and Dr. William Albrecht, Walters used the magazine, and later books and conferences, to advocate for sustainable agriculture that prioritized soil health and natural processes. Acres U.S.A. provided a platform for these ideas and helped to popularize alternative methods like cover cropping and integrated livestock management.

Though the agricultural landscape still relies heavily on conventional methods, Acres U.S.A. has been instrumental in the growing movement toward regenerative agriculture. By disseminating knowledge and supporting eco-conscious farmers, the company continues to champion sustainable practices through its publications, conferences, and online resources, contributing to a shift toward a more ecologically sound approach to farming.

Find Out More About Acres U.S.A.

Soil Nutrition Handbook
Understanding soil & soil reports

The information in this book is true and complete to the best of our knowledge. All recommendations are made without guarantee on the part of the authors and Acres U.S.A. The authors and publisher disclaim any liability in connection with the use or misuse of this information.

PO Box 351
Viroqua, WI 54665 U.S.A.
512-892-4400
info@acresusa.com • www.acresusa.com

Printed in the United States of America

ISBN 978-1-60173-994-0:

Contents

About Us

RAD RESTORATION AGRICULTURE DEVELOPMENT

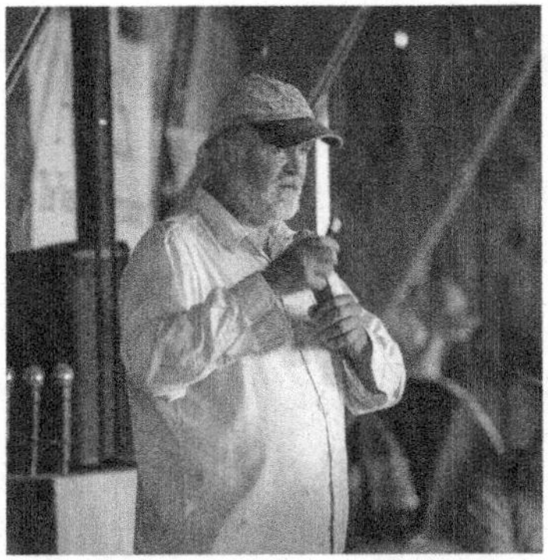

Mark Shepard

Mark Shepard is the CEO of Restoration Agriculture Development and the Forest Agriculture Nursery. He runs New Forest Farms, a 110-acre perennial agricultural savanna that is one of the first of its kind in the USA. He has designed and installed agroforestry systems across North America, Europe, and Africa for over twenty years. He is the author of the award-winning and Amazon best-selling book *Restoration Agriculture: Real-world Permaculture for Farmers* and *Water for ANY Farm*, both published by Acres U.S.A.

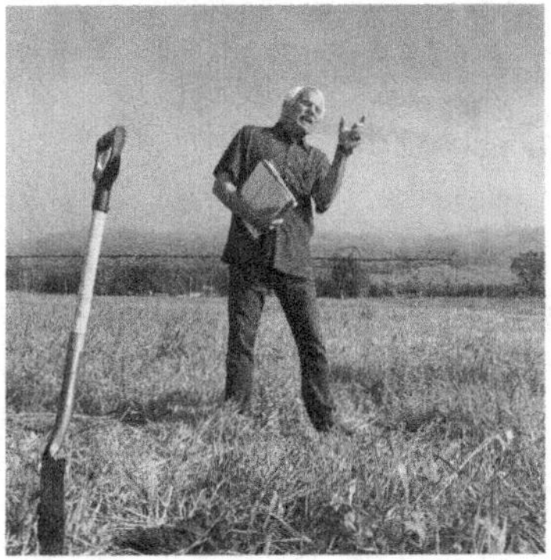

Gary Zimmer

Gary Zimmer is known as the father of biological farming. He and his family own Otter Creek Organic Farm—a 1500-acre farm in the Spring Green, Wisconsin area. He has developed an extreme soil-building farming system with highly mineralized soils—one year in rye/clover cover crops and the next year in corn. Gary is the founder of Midwestern BioAg, is presently promoting carbon-based fertility systems by building designer compost, and is the author of three books and numerous articles on soils and livestock nutrition. He holds a bachelor's degree from the University of Wisconsin-Madison and a master's degree in Dairy Nutrition from the University of Hawaii.

"This country will not be a good place for any of us to live in unless we make it a good place for all of us to live in."

-Theodore Roosevelt

How to Use This Handbook

Understanding Your Report

Not all of us have a lifetime of experience reading and interpreting cation-balancing soil test results. The results from most university tests show how much nitrogen, phosphorus, and potassium are required to reach target yield levels. On the standard soil test, calcium is mostly looked at as a way of raising pH. Not all of us want to spend the time and energy it takes to read the Albrecht Papers (available through Acres U.S.A.) and memorize all of the principles behind soil mineral balancing. This condensed handbook is a summary of the most significant information—quick, sound, immediately applicable advice for farmers and ranchers.

The core principle of soil mineral balancing is that soil health and fertility are dependent on balanced ratios of mineral cations in the soil. Excessive amounts of one mineral can result in apparent deficiencies in another. For example, excess magnesium can prevent the proper uptake of calcium. This leads to symptoms of calcium deficiency even if there is enough calcium in the soil.

A well-balanced soil leads to optimized soil aggregation, improved tilth, rapid and extensive root penetration, good water infiltration, and long-term crop productivity. Short-term additions of N-P-K fertilizers may give short-term yield boosts but eventually lead to mineral imbalances. Out-of-balance minerals lead to out-of-balance soil life, which leads to crops that are more susceptible to pests, diseases, and environmental extremes.

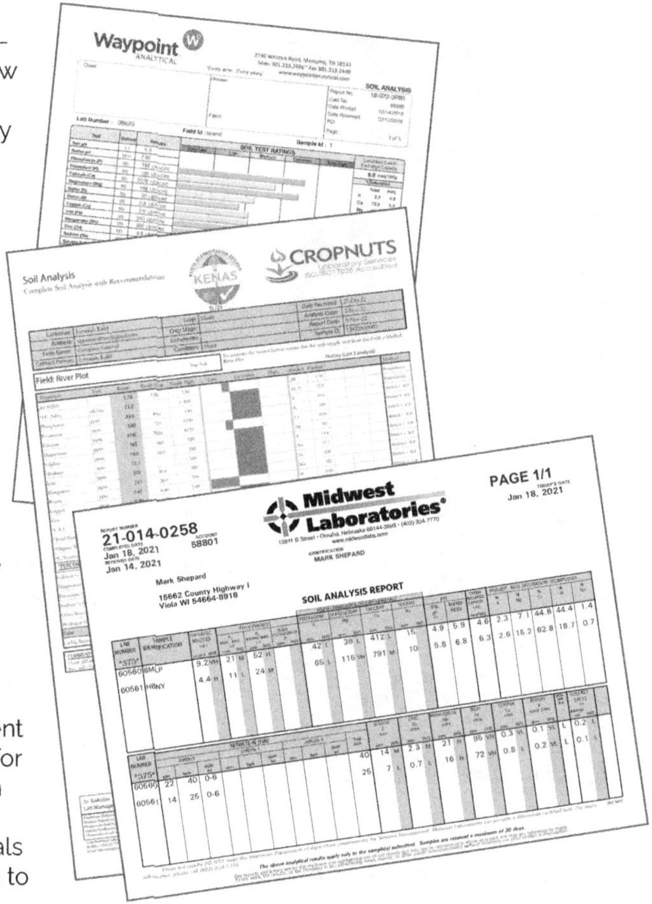

The numbers in this guide are based off Midwest Labs. If you use a different lab, their numbers may be somewhat different, but what you are looking for are excesses and deficiencies. Add whatever is short. If the levels are high enough, there is no need to correct the soil. Which inputs and how much of them you use will vary based on area, budget, and crops grown. Minerals perform best within a carbon/biological cyle, so it's essential to add them to manures and compost and when growing cover crops.

Soil Life and Nutrient Balance

In order to grow high yields of healthy crops, plants need sunshine, water, and mineral nutrients linked with biological carbon. A soil test is necessary to discover which mineral nutrients are actually present in your soil. This allows a farmer or rancher to know what to strategically add to increase soil health, crop yields, and crop quality. Well-balanced mineral nutrients result in healthy soil life, healthy plants and animals, and healthy people.

Soil testing allows us to make intelligent soil corrections. It may take a long time to correct soils that are far out of balance. Whatever minerals the soil doesn't provide will need to be added to the soil or the crop as fertilizer if you want healthy, nutrient-rich crops. To know what our crops need, we need to know—not just guess—what's in the soil. Ample amounts of a compost that is deficient in critical minerals will not supply those minerals to the crop. Adding the "right" soil biology to make minerals available will not help if those minerals are not present.

Soil testing provides a useful guide by telling us what kind of soil we are dealing with and what its limiting factors are. It doesn't necessarily measure plant availability of minerals, but it tells us what building blocks we have to work with. Improving soil biology makes these minerals available to plant roots.

Five Lessons from Soil Testing

1. ***What type of soil is it?*** Organic matter, cation exchange capacity (CEC), and pH tell us this.
2. ***Phosphorus (P) and potassium (K) levels.*** These are important elements, so most agronomists will recommend adding more even if the soil test is high, based on crop removal. Why not replace ALL minerals removed, not just P and K? We can measure removal by repeating soil tests on a regular basis—every year at first, then every two or three years as the system matures.
3. ***Calcium (Ca) and magnesium (Mg).*** Both the total levels and ratio between these two elements are extremely important.
4. ***Trace elements (Zn, Cu, Mn, Fe, etc.).*** These are extremely important for plant health and performance, although they are needed only in small amounts.
5. ***Uniformity.*** This gives clues to help decide which minerals to adjust first.

Ecological Farming/Ranching Goals

- Improved mineral balance and soil life.
- Improved crop performance and quality. Quality soil leads to quality crops and higher yields.
- Healthy soil grows healthy crops. Healthy crops lead to healthy livestock.
- Improved yield and quality leads to rapid weight gain and lowered veterinary and feed bills. Lower costs with higher gains lead to bigger profit margins.

Essential Nutrients

Although scientists continue to debate how many plant nutrients are essential, most agree that at least seventeen nutrients are critical for plant growth.

Non-mineral nutrients: Carbon (C), hydrogen (H), and oxygen (O). These are the building blocks used by the plant during photosynthesis to make glucose.

Macronutrients: Nitrogen (N), phosphorus (P), and potassium (K). These are needed in large amounts and are the primary ingredients of fertilizers.

Secondary Macronutrients: Calcium (Ca) and sulfur (S). Although most large-scale chemical-ag operations consider these nutrients to be "secondary," ecological farmers recognize that these nutrients are essential for almost every cellular process and are needed in quantities almost as large as nitrogen.

Micronutrients/trace elements: Zinc (Zn), manganese (Mn), iron (Fe), copper (Cu), boron (B), molybdenum (Mo), chlorine (Cl), and nickel (Ni). Other nutrients, such as iodine, are found in plants and plant products, but scientists disagree on how essential they are for plant growth.

Well-Balanced Soil

Phosphorus	50 ppm
Potassium	3–5 % saturation
Magnesium	12–15 % saturation
Calcium	70–80 % saturation
Sulfur	50 ppm
N:S Ratio	10 : 1
Ca:K Ratio	10 : 1
Ca:Mg Ratio	5 : 1
pH Level	6.7–6.9

Medium (3-6%) Organic Matter

Adequate Trace Elements

Benefits of Balance

Solid-stemmed alfalfa

Good dry-down and keeping quality

High sugar content

Good mineral balance

Healthy animals

Low weather stress

High yield

Fewer weed problems

A Barrel of Nutrients

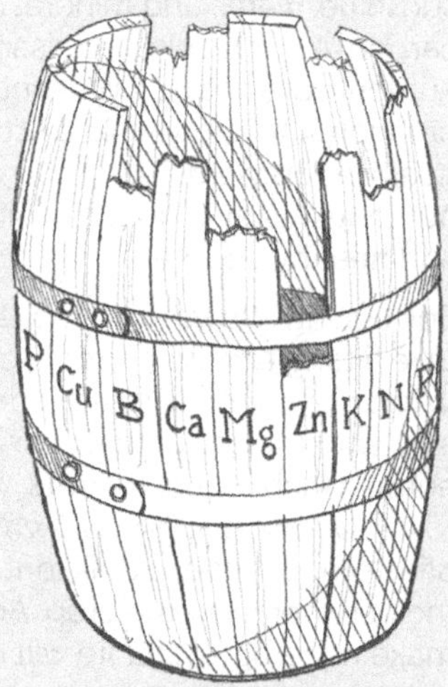

The productivity of a soil can never be greater than the essential nutrient in least supply.

Organic Matter

Organic matter is the portion of the soil that consists of plant or animal tissue in various stages of decomposition. These materials provide plant nutrients, microorganism habitat, and soil structure as they circulate through the farm ecosystem.

Organic matter can be grouped into three major types:

1. **Plant Residues** and living microbial biomass
2. **Detritus**—soil organic matter which is actively being eaten
3. **Humus**—stable soil organic matter

SOIL ANALYSIS REPORT

LAB NUMBER *375*	SAMPLE IDENTIFICATION	ORGANIC MATTER L.O.I. percent	ORGANIC MATTER RATE	PHOSPHORUS P1 (WEAK BRAY) 1:7 ppm	P1 RATE	PHOSPHORUS P2 (STRONG BRAY) 1:7 ppm	P2 RATE	OLSEN BICARBONATE P ppm	OLSEN RATE	POTASSIUM K ppm	K RATE	MAGNESIUM Mg ppm	Mg RATE	CALCIUM Ca ppm	Ca RATE	SODIUM Na ppm	Na RATE	pH SOIL pH 1:1	pH BUFFER INDEX	CATION EXCHANGE CAPACITY C.E.C. meq/100g	PERCENT BASE SATURATION (COMPUTED) % K	% Mg	% Ca	% H	% Na
60560	BMLP	9.2	VH	21	M	52	H			42	L	39	L	412	L	15		4.9	5.9	4.6	2.3	7.1	44.8	44.4	1.4
60561	HBNY	4.4	H	11	L	24	M			65	L	115	VH	791	M	10		5.8	6.8	6.3	2.6	15.2	62.8	18.7	0.7

(POTASSIUM, MAGNESIUM, CALCIUM, SODIUM: NEUTRAL AMMONIUM ACETATE(EXCHANGEABLE))

LAB NUMBER *375*	NITRATE-N (FIA) SURFACE ppm	SURFACE lbs/A	SURFACE depth (in)	SUBSOIL 1 ppm	SUBSOIL 1 lbs/A	SUBSOIL 1 depth (in)	SUBSOIL 2 ppm	SUBSOIL 2 lbs/A	SUBSOIL 2 depth (in)	Total lbs/A	SULFUR S ICAP ppm	S RATE	ZINC Zn DTPA ppm	Zn RATE	MANGANESE Mn DTPA ppm	Mn RATE	IRON Fe DTPA ppm	Fe RATE	COPPER Cu DTPA ppm	Cu RATE	BORON B SORB. DTPA ppm	B RATE	EXCESS LIME RATE	SOLUBLE SALTS 1:1 mmhos/cm	SOLUBLE SALTS RATE
60560	22	40	0-6							40	14	M	2.3	M	21	H	95	VH	0.3	VL	0.1	VL	L	0.2	L
60561	14	25	0-6							25	7	L	0.7	L	16	H	72	VH	0.8	L	0.2	VL	L	0.1	L

Organic Matter

Cycling Organic Matter

Essential Nutrients

Essential Nutrients for Plant Growth

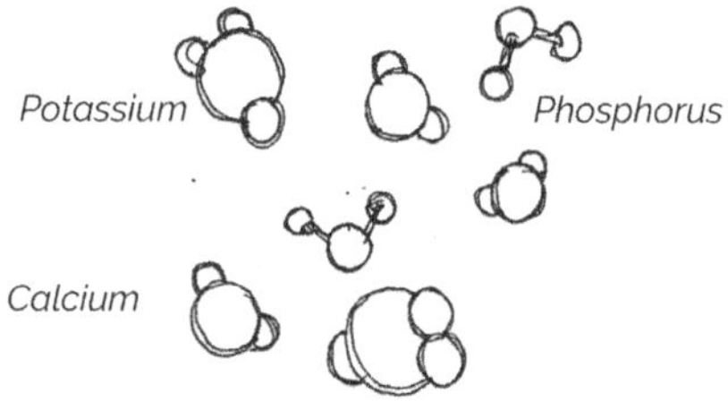

Taken Up

Plants combine atmospheric carbon, water, and essential plant nutrients to create raw organic matter such as cellulose and lignin. Soil animals consume raw organic matter and are in turn eaten by larger animals.

Raw Organic Matter

Plant residue, leaf litter, animal manures, etc.

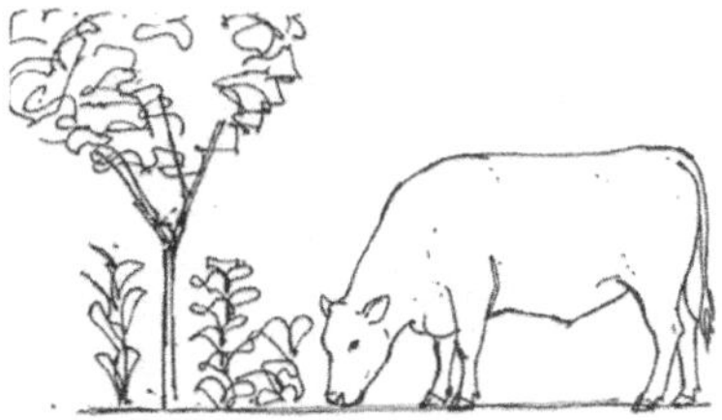

Decomposed

Soil detritus is eaten for energy and nutrition by detritivores such as fungi, bacteria, arthropods, worms, beetles, etc. These creatures break it down into smaller and smaller pieces, eventually reducing it to essential mineral nutrients.

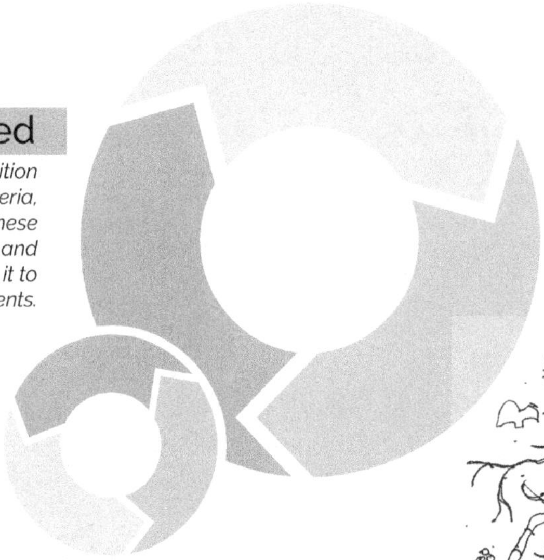

Dropped

Plant roots exude simple sugars back into the soil. Plant material falls to the surface as litter, and dead roots slough off beneath the soil. Animals consume nutrients and then redeposit them as manure and urine.

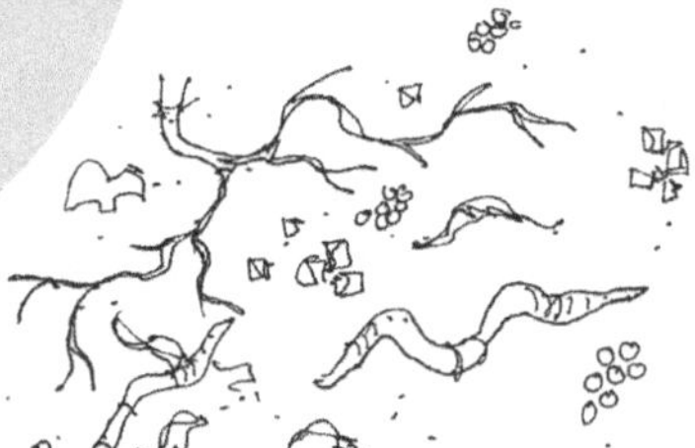

Humus

A semi-stable soil carbon matrix

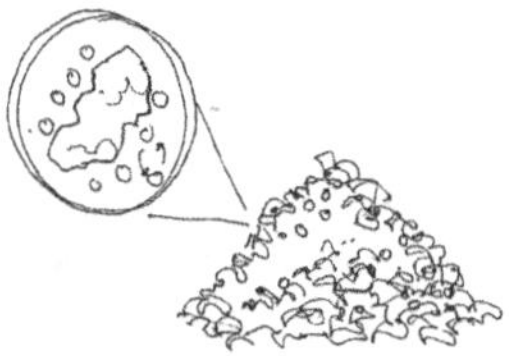

Soil Detritus

Being eaten by microbes, fungi, worms, etc.

Humus

In Balance	Out of Balance
Active biological life	No life; no earthy smell
Reduced erosion	Erosion
Good tilth; loose soil	Crusted, cloddy, hard-to-work soil
Good water intake and retention	Waterlogging; poor drainage
Large root systems and no hardpan	Hardpan
Fewer weeds	High weed pressure
Fewer pests and diseases	Insect and disease problems
Rapid organic matter decomposition	Poor organic matter decomposition
Many earthworms	Little or no earthworm activity
Fewer chemicals needed	More fertilizers/chemicals needed

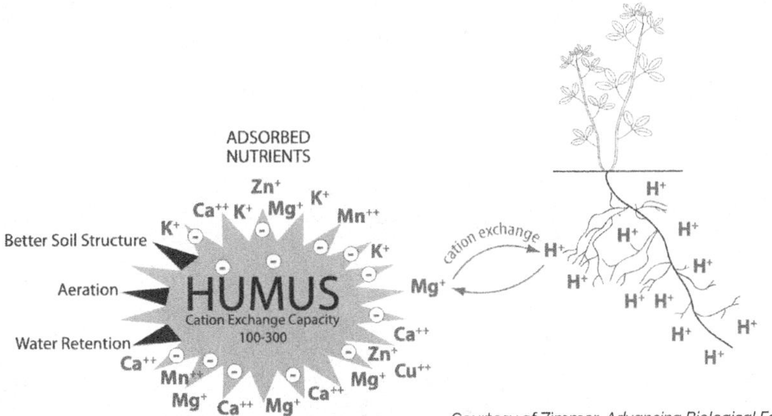

Courtesy of Zimmer, *Advancing Biological Farming*, pg. 201

A Word on Carbon

Carbon is an essential plant nutrient, fertilizer, and growth stimulant. It is the building block of carbohydrates, proteins, and oils. The energy stored in the bonds between carbon and hydrogen fuels everything from microscopic cellular processes to ecosystems and civilizations. Carbon provides the skeletal framework for the body of every living being. It attaches to the minerals that are essential for life and growth. It holds water and nutrients like a sponge and provides habitat for soil life.

Cation Exchange Capacity

Cation Exchange

Plant roots can access nutrients from the soil through a process known as **cation exchange**. During this process, positively charged nutrient particles transfer from the soil to plant roots in exchange for positively charged hydrogen molecules exuded by plant roots. This results in nutrients moving from the soil into the plants.

Roots in the Soil

Physical and chemical characteristics of the soil determine how many nutrients can be stored in the soil and exchanged with plants.

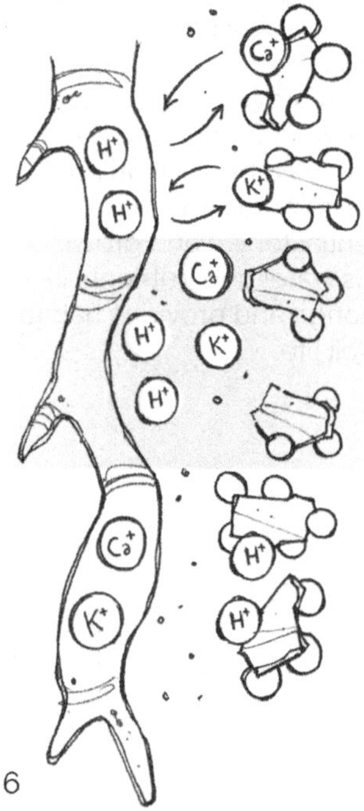

1: *Negatively charged soil particles hold positively charged cations/nutrients*

2: *Plant roots exchange hydrogen cations for essential nutrients they cannot produce themselves*

3: *New nutrients enter the soil in the form of raw organic matter, manufactured soil amendments, or dissolution/chelation of parent material*

Cation Exchange Capacity

Cation exchange capacity (CEC) is a measure of a soil's ability to supply nutrients for plant uptake. CEC measures the total negative charges within the soil that adsorb plant nutrient cations such as calcium (Ca^{2+}), magnesium (Mg^{2+}), and potassium (K^+). Three primary factors determine the CEC of a soil: particle size, soil pH, and the amount of organic matter present.

Low C.E.C. .... High C.E.C.

Particle Size

Low C.E.C.	High C.E.C.
Large soil particles (sandy soil)	*Small soil particles (clay soil)*
Low surface area	*High surface area*
Less potential for exchange	*More potential for exchange*

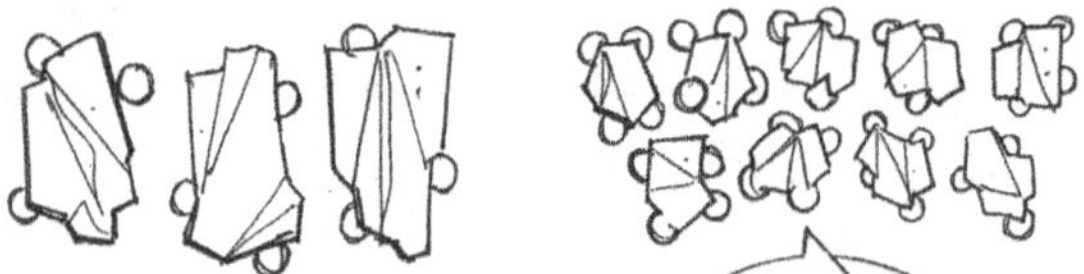

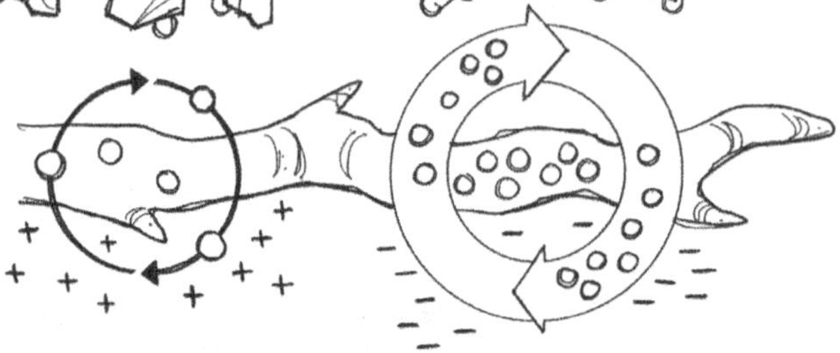

Soil PH

Low C.E.C.	High C.E.C.
Low pH reading (acidic soil)	*High pH reading (basic soil)*
Too many positive charges	*Ample negative charges*
Less potential for exchange	*More potential for exchange*

Organic Matter, particularly Humus, improves CEC

Cation Exchange Capacity

Because cation exchange capacity is a measure of the soil's ability to store and release essential nutrients, it is an important indicator of the soil's potential for crop production. Without knowing the CEC, it is difficult to make recommendations for improving soil conditions.

As a measurement of a soil's ability to hold and supply nutrients to plants, CEC is a key indicator of soil fertility. A higher CEC will yield more produce per acre, and well-managed soil can retain a high CEC for many seasons.

SOIL ANALYSIS REPORT

LAB NUMBER *375*	SAMPLE IDENTIFICATION	ORGANIC MATTER L.O.I. percent	RATE	PHOSPHORUS P1 (WEAK BRAY) 1:7 ppm	RATE	PHOSPHORUS P2 (STRONG BRAY) 1:7 ppm	RATE	PHOSPHORUS OLSEN BICARBONATE P ppm	RATE	NEUTRAL AMMONIUM ACETATE (EXCHANGEABLE) POTASSIUM K ppm	RATE	MAGNESIUM Mg ppm	RATE	CALCIUM Ca ppm	RATE	SODIUM Na ppm	RATE	pH SOIL pH 1:1	pH BUFFER INDEX	CATION EXCHANGE CAPACITY C.E.C. meq/100g	PERCENT BASE SATURATION (COMPUTED) % K	% Mg	% Ca	% H	% Na
60560	BMLP	9.2	VH	21	M	52	H			42	L	39	L	412	L	15		4.9	5.9	**4.6**	2.3	7.1	44.8	44.4	1.4
60561	HBNY	4.4	H	11	L	24	M			65	L	115	VH	791	M	10		5.8	6.8	**6.3**	2.6	15.2	62.8	18.7	0.7

LAB NUMBER *375*	NITRATE-N (FIA) SURFACE ppm	SURFACE lbs/A	SURFACE depth (in)	SUBSOIL 1 ppm	SUBSOIL 1 lbs/A	SUBSOIL 1 depth (in)	SUBSOIL 2 ppm	SUBSOIL 2 lbs/A	SUBSOIL 2 depth (in)	Total lbs/A	SULFUR S ICAP ppm	RATE	ZINC Zn DTPA ppm	RATE	MANGANESE Mn DTPA ppm	RATE	IRON Fe DTPA ppm	RATE	COPPER Cu DTPA ppm	RATE	BORON B SORB. DTPA ppm	RATE	EXCESS LIME RATE	SOLUBLE SALTS 1:1 mmhos/cm	RATE	
60560	22	40	0-6							40	14	M	2.3	M	21	H	95	VH	0.3	VL	0.1	VL	L	0.2	L	
60561	14	25	0-6							25	7	L	0.7	L	16	H	72	VH	0.8	L	0.2	VL	L	0.1	L	

Base Saturation

Percent Base Saturation

Percent base saturation is the relative amount of specific cations (positively charged ions, or bases) held on soil colloids, expressed as a percent of total cation exchange capacity (CEC). The desired levels are 70 to 85 percent calcium, 12 to 18 percent magnesium, 3 to 5 percent potassium, less than 5 percent hydrogen, and less than 1 percent sodium. Soils in arid regions tend to have high levels of sodium.

In a low-CEC soil, even if the proportions of nutrient cations are ideal, the soil may not be able to provide them to the crop in sufficient quantities. The producer will have to supplement low-CEC soils with extra fertilizer.

Excessively high levels of hydrogen and sodium limit plant growth, as do shortages or excesses of other cations. Percent base saturation lets us know how much amendment is necessary to bring nutrient ratios into a range more favorable to plant growth.

High levels of soil hydrogen (H) increase soil acidity. High levels of soil sodium (Na) cause soil aggregates to fall apart. Pore spaces get filled in and "cemented," limiting available water, nutrients, and root penetration.

CEC	ppm Potassium 3.2% base saturation	ppm Magnesium 15% base saturation	ppm Calcium 75% base saturation
4.0	50*	72*	600*
5.0	62*	90*	750*
6.0	75*	108*	900*
7.0	87*	126	1,050*
8.0	100*	144	1,200*
9.0	112*	162	1,350
10.0	125	180	1,500
11.0	137	198	1,650
12.0	150	216	1,800
13.0	162	234	1,950
14.0	175	252	2,100
15.0	187	270	2,250
16.0	200	288	2,400
17.0	212	306	2,550
18.0	225	324	2,700
19.0	237	342	2,850
20.0	250	360	3,000

Formulas: For potassium: 780 x CEC x 3.2 ÷ 200 =
For magnesium: 240 x CEC x 15 ÷ 200 =
For calcium: 400 x CEC x 75 ÷ 200 =
** Low-CEC soils may need higher levels of potassium, calcium, and magnesium than given in this table to produce high-quality crops.*

What Is Soil pH?

Soil pH is a measurement of the concentration of hydrogen ions in the soil, expressed as the negative logarithm of the hydrogen ion concentration. With every whole number change in the pH, there is a tenfold change in hydrogen ion concentration. A pH of 5.8, for example, is ten times more acidic than 6.8, and 4.8 is one hundred times more acidic than 6.8.

Most of the cation exchange capacity in a fertile soil is filled with cations that are plant nutrients, like calcium, magnesium, potassium, and ammonium. As roots absorb nutrient cations, they exchange them with hydrogen ions. As hydrogen accumulates over time, the soil becomes more acidic and the pH drops. Below a pH of 5, aluminum ions are released from clay particles, which contributes even more to soil acidity.

Plant nutrient availability varies with pH. Some nutrients are less available at low pH (acid), and others are less available at high pH (alkaline). Soil pH also affects the activity of beneficial soil microbes. Bacteria and actinomycetes prefer more alkaline soils, while fungi do best in acid conditions. In general, an acid soil is a low-fertility soil.

Nutrient Availability and pH

For plants to take up the nutrients required for growth, those nutrients need to be present in the soil at certain levels. Larger root systems, better soil biology, and better soil structure can improve plant nutrient uptake, but adequate amounts of those nutrients actually need to be present in the soil. If you provide all minerals sufficient levels of all essential minerals, you will balance the soil and greatly improve crop performance. There are also ratios between specific minerals—like calcium to magnesium—which affect mineral uptake, soil structure, and crop performance.

If the soil has extremes that are impossible to correct—like high magnesium or high pH—it is beneficial to hook your minerals to a carbon source like humus or compost before applying them to the soil.

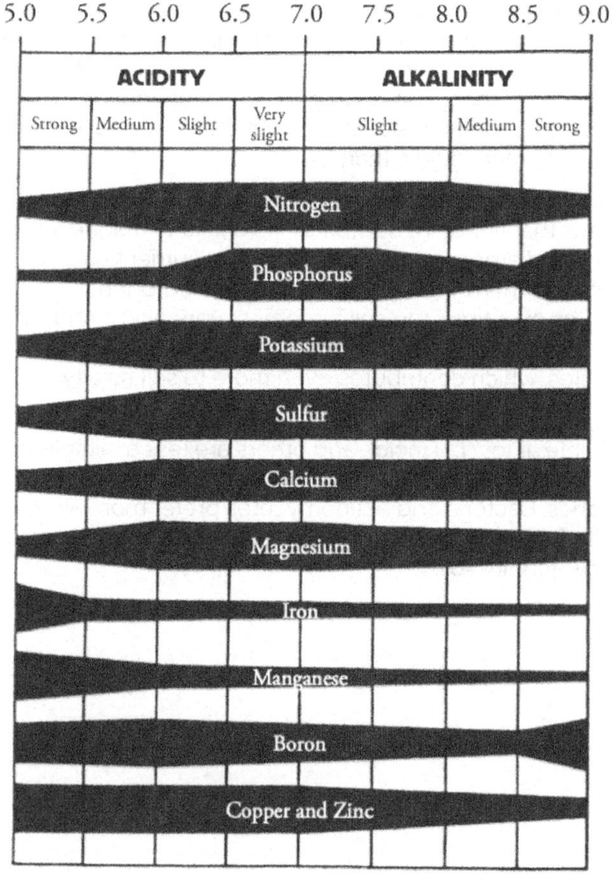

Availability of Elements to Plants at Different pH Levels for Typical Soils

The Elements in Soil

The important nutrients for plant development are of low atomic mass. They create three apparent clusters: one in the alkali and alkaline metals, one in the transition metals, and one in the non-metals and metalloids (clustered around carbon).

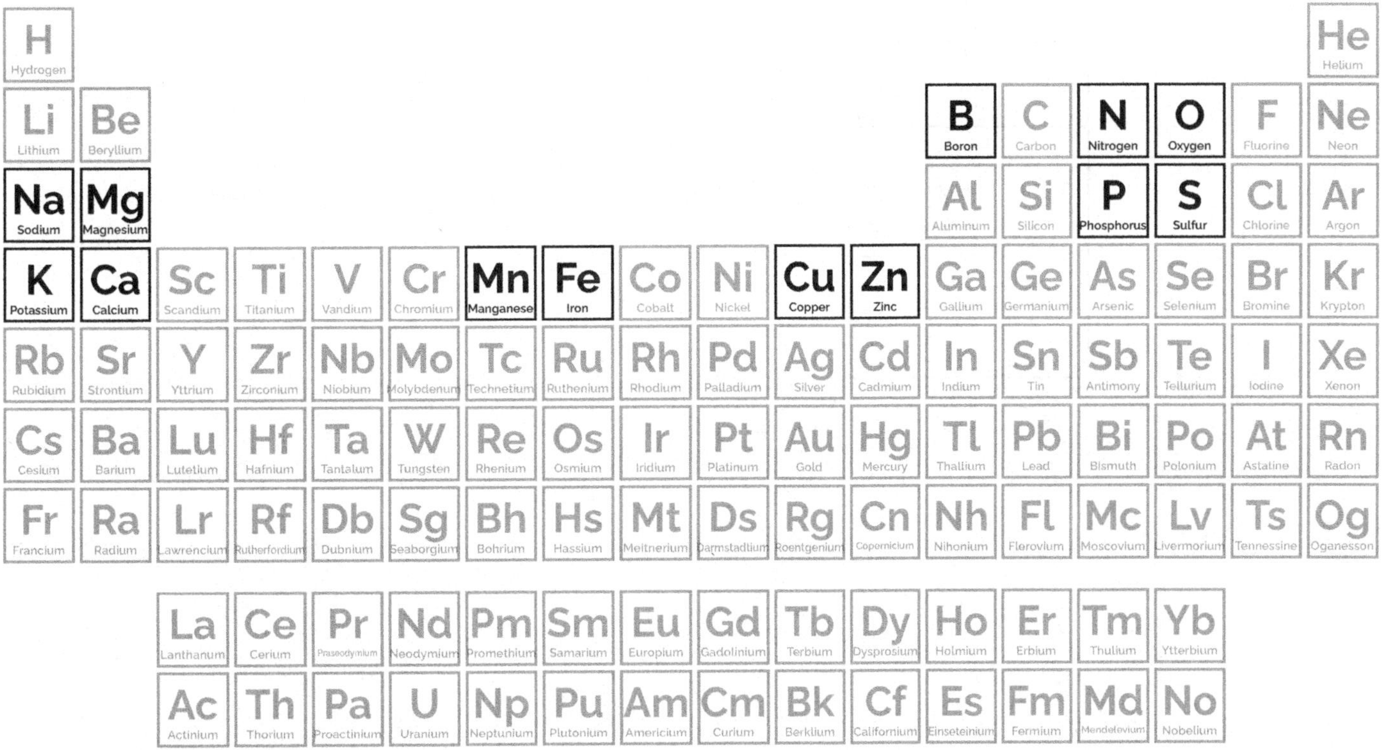

Phosphorus

Phosphorus is a constituent of plant cells which is essential for cell division and growing tip development. For this reason, it is vital for seedlings and young plants. Phosphorus is vital for energy transfer within plants because it assists in photosynthesis, transformation of sugars and starches, and nutrient movement.

SOIL ANALYSIS REPORT

LAB NUMBER *375*	SAMPLE IDENTIFICATION	ORGANIC MATTER L.O.I. percent	RATE	PHOSPHORUS P_1 (WEAK BRAY) 1:7 ppm	RATE	PHOSPHORUS P_2 (STRONG BRAY) 1:7 ppm	RATE	PHOSPHORUS OLSEN BICARBONATE P ppm	RATE	NEUTRAL AMMONIUM ACETATE (EXCHANGEABLE) POTASSIUM K ppm	RATE	MAGNESIUM Mg ppm	RATE	CALCIUM Ca ppm	RATE	SODIUM Na ppm	RATE	pH SOIL pH 1:1	pH BUFFER INDEX	CATION EXCHANGE CAPACITY C.E.C. meq/100g	PERCENT BASE SATURATION (COMPUTED) % K	% Mg	% Ca	% H	% Na
60560	BMLP	9.2	VH	21	M	52	H			42	L	39	L	412	L	15		4.9	5.9	4.6	2.3	7.1	44.8	44.4	1.4
60561	HBNY	4.4	H	11	L	24	M			65	L	115	VH	791	M	10		5.8	6.8	6.3	2.6	15.2	62.8	18.7	0.7

LAB NUMBER *375*	NITRATE-N (FIA) SURFACE ppm	SURFACE lbs/A	SURFACE depth (in)	SUBSOIL 1 ppm	SUBSOIL 1 lbs/A	SUBSOIL 1 depth (in)	SUBSOIL 2 ppm	SUBSOIL 2 lbs/A	SUBSOIL 2 depth (in)	Total lbs/A	SULFUR S ICAP ppm	RATE	ZINC Zn DTPA ppm	RATE	MANGANESE Mn DTPA ppm	RATE	IRON Fe DTPA ppm	RATE	COPPER Cu DTPA ppm	RATE	BORON B SORB. DTPA ppm	RATE	EXCESS LIME RATE	SOLUBLE SALTS 1:1 mmhos/cm	RATE	
60560	22	40	0-6							40	14	M	2.3	M	21	H	95	VH	0.3	VL	0.1	VL	L	0.2	L	
60561	14	25	0-6							25	7	L	0.7	L	16	H	72	VH	0.8	L	0.2	VL	L	0.1	L	

Phosphorus

15 30.974

P

Phosphorus

On farm after farm, phosphorus uptake is a major limiting factor. Start balancing a soil with calcium and phosphorus. Higher soil levels than most agronomists recommend are okay, because there needs to be enough for a high-yielding, healthy crop. Excess phosphorus will not create apparent deficiencies in other minerals. Higher soil phosphorus may require more zinc use, but a high uptake affects plant health and performance. Phosphorus is a biological mineral with a strong negative charge. It ties up easily with iron and aluminum in low-pH soils. At a high pH, it binds with calcium. Phosphorus as a soil corrective is best applied with a carbon source like manure, compost, or humates. Using natural sources like rock phosphate ensures a long-term supply that can be released by active soil life. A soil test of P1 at 50 ppm and P2 at 100 with a neutral pH is a nice place to be.

Benefits

- Fast and vigorous growth
- Good and early root growth
- Grain development and quality
- Hastens maturity
- Increased nitrogen uptake
- Increased mineral content
- Higher sugar in plant
- Energy release in cells
- Cell division and enlargement
- Photosynthesis
- Contained in cell DNA

Ideal Levels

- P1 (weak Bray)—50 ppm
- P2 (strong Bray)—100 ppm

Best Sources

- Poultry manure
- Bat/bird guano
- Phosphate rock
- Monoammonium phosphate (MAP) 11-52-0 or 10-50-0

Comments

- We use MAP because it has a low pH of 5, is more available, and has a low ammonium content.
- Avoid using diammonium phosphate (DAP) because it has a toxic pH of 11 and a high ammonium content, which harms root development by burning off the root hairs.
- On farm after farm, phosphorus uptake is a major limiting factor. When balancing a soil, the best place to start is with calcium and phosphorus. Higher soil phosphorus may require more zinc use, but a high uptake of phosphorus positively affects plant health and performance. Phosphorus is a biological mineral with a strong negative charge. It ties up easily in low pH soils, especially with iron and aluminum. At a high pH, it ties up with calcium.
- Using manure or rock phosphate added to compost or mixed with humates greatly improves availability. The nutrients are then already "hooked" to carbon and can't be tied up.

Potassium

Potassium helps plants grow rigid and tall and improves their resistance to weather variation by helping to regulate the opening and closing of stomata. Potassium is also associated with the movement of water, nutrients, and carbohydrates in plant tissue.

SOIL ANALYSIS REPORT

LAB NUMBER *375*	SAMPLE IDENTIFICATION	ORGANIC MATTER L.O.I. percent	RATE	PHOSPHORUS P1 (WEAK BRAY) 1:7 ppm	RATE	PHOSPHORUS P2 (STRONG BRAY) 1:7 ppm	RATE	PHOSPHORUS OLSEN BICARBONATE P ppm	RATE	NEUTRAL AMMONIUM ACETATE (EXCHANGEABLE): POTASSIUM K ppm	RATE	MAGNESIUM Mg ppm	RATE	CALCIUM Ca ppm	RATE	SODIUM Na ppm	RATE	pH SOIL pH	pH BUFFER INDEX	CATION EXCHANGE CAPACITY C.E.C. meq/100g	PERCENT BASE SATURATION (COMPUTED) % K	% Mg	% Ca	% H	% Na
60560	BMLP	9.2	VH	21	M	52	H			42	L	39	L	412	L	15		4.9	5.9	4.6	2.3	7.1	44.8	44.4	1.4
60561	HBNY	4.4	H	11	L	24	M			65	L	115	VH	791	M	10		5.8	6.8	6.3	2.6	15.2	62.8	18.7	0.7

LAB NUMBER *375*	NITRATE-N (FIA) SURFACE ppm	SURFACE lbs/A	SURFACE depth (in)	SUBSOIL 1 ppm	SUBSOIL 1 lbs/A	SUBSOIL 1 depth (in)	SUBSOIL 2 ppm	SUBSOIL 2 lbs/A	SUBSOIL 2 depth (in)	Total lbs/A	SULFUR S ICAP ppm	RATE	ZINC Zn DTPA ppm	RATE	MANGANESE Mn DTPA ppm	RATE	IRON Fe DTPA ppm	RATE	COPPER Cu DTPA ppm	RATE	BORON B SORB. DTPA ppm	RATE	EXCESS LIME RATE	SOLUBLE SALTS 1:1 mmhos/cm	RATE
60560	22	40	0-6							40	14	M	2.3	M	21	H	95	VH	0.3	VL	0.1	VL	L	0.2	L
60561	14	25	0-6							25	7	L	0.7	L	16	H	72	VH	0.8	L	0.2	VL	L	0.1	L

Potassium

19 39.098

K

Potassium

Benefits

- Yield potential
- Stalk strength; lodging resistance
- Winter hardiness
- Protein production
- Carbohydrate production; sugar translocation
- Enzyme functions
- Cell division

Ideal Levels

- 125–175 ppm
- More than 3–5% of total exchangeable nutrients

Best Sources

- Organic matter (decomposing sawdust, straw, and hay mulch)
- Animal manure
- Compost
- Granite dust
- Kelp
- Termite mound soil
- Potassium sulfate (0-0-50-17S)
- K-Mag (0-0-22-22S-11Mg)

Comments

- Potassium levels should never fall below 100 ppm, regardless of CEC
- Excess potassium can cause problems
- Potassium chloride (0-0-60) is the cheapest potassium source but should be used with caution because of its chlorine content. If you must apply it, a fall application is best.
- Granite dust is extremely slow-release and requires healthy soil life. Soils on granite bedrock frequently have enough potassium and need no additions.
- Potassium is a monovalent (single-charge) cation, so it bonds weakly to the soil, is more soluble, and is easier to get into a plant. It's an important nutrient, but over-application can cause problems and interfere with the uptake of other minerals.
- Potassium is a highly soluble mineral and easily supplied; spoon-feed it.

Magnesium

As iron is the central element in human blood, magnesium is the central element in the chlorophyll molecule. It is instrumental for collecting energy from the sun. Proper magnesium levels keep leaves a healthy green color.

SOIL ANALYSIS REPORT

LAB NUMBER *375*	SAMPLE IDENTIFICATION	ORGANIC MATTER L.O.I. percent	ORGANIC MATTER RATE	PHOSPHORUS P_1 (WEAK BRAY) 1:7 ppm	P_1 RATE	PHOSPHORUS P_2 (STRONG BRAY) 1:7 ppm	P_2 RATE	OLSEN BICARBONATE P ppm	OLSEN RATE	POTASSIUM K ppm	K RATE	MAGNESIUM Mg ppm	Mg RATE	CALCIUM Ca ppm	Ca RATE	SODIUM Na ppm	Na RATE	pH SOIL pH 1:1	pH BUFFER INDEX	CATION EXCHANGE CAPACITY C.E.C. meq/100g	PERCENT BASE SATURATION (COMPUTED) % K	% Mg	% Ca	% H	% Na
60560	BMLP	9.2	VH	21	M	52	H			42	L	39	L	412	L	15		4.9	5.9	4.6	2.3	7.1	44.8	44.4	1.4
60561	HBNY	4.4	H	11	L	24	M			65	L	115	VH	791	M	10		5.8	6.8	6.3	2.6	15.2	62.8	18.7	0.7

(Potassium, Magnesium, Calcium, Sodium: NEUTRAL AMMONIUM ACETATE (EXCHANGEABLE))

LAB NUMBER *375*	NITRATE-N (FIA) SURFACE ppm	SURFACE lbs/A	SURFACE depth (in)	SUBSOIL 1 ppm	SUBSOIL 1 lbs/A	SUBSOIL 1 depth (in)	SUBSOIL 2 ppm	SUBSOIL 2 lbs/A	SUBSOIL 2 depth (in)	Total lbs/A	SULFUR S ICAP ppm	S RATE	ZINC Zn DTPA ppm	Zn RATE	MANGANESE Mn DTPA ppm	Mn RATE	IRON Fe DTPA ppm	Fe RATE	COPPER Cu DTPA ppm	Cu RATE	BORON B SORB. DTPA ppm	B RATE	EXCESS LIME RATE	SOLUBLE SALTS 1:1 mmhos/cm	SOLUBLE SALTS RATE
60560	22	40	0-6							40	14	M	2.3	M	21	H	95	VH	0.3	VL	0.1	VL	L	0.2	L
60561	14	25	0-6							25	7	L	0.7	L	16	H	72	VH	0.8	L	0.2	VL	L	0.1	L

Magnesium

12 24.305
Mg
Magnesium

Benefits

- Key element in chlorophyll
- Protein production
- Enzyme functions
- Energy release in cells
- Phosphorus uptake
- Oil formation
- Starch translocation

Best Sources

- Magnesium sulfate (9% Mg, 12% S)
- K-Mag (0-0-22-22S-11Mg)

Ideal Levels

- 100–500 ppm
- 15–20% of total exchangeable cations

Comments

- Excess magnesium can cause the following problems:
- Tight soil
- Hard-to-balance soil
- Tied-up potassium
- Reduced nitrogen utilization
- Magnesium is one of the hardest minerals to get into a plant because it is tightly held and is also directly competitive with potassium. Just because the soil test says you have Mg doesn't mean it's getting into the plant. Most magnesium in the soil is in the form of magnesium carbonate, which is not soluble. Magnesium sulfate is highly soluble, so if the soil level is sufficient and you are not overdoing K, apply some sulfur. Having a plant test high in Mg and P is a great indicator of plant and soil health and performance.

Calcium

The Trucker of All Nutrients

Calcium promotes the growth of plant tissues and membranes and strengthens cell walls. This is especially important for the development of root systems, which uptake various nutrients. Calcium is also one of the factors that determines the pH level of the soil, which has to have the right balance of acidity and alkalinity.

SOIL ANALYSIS REPORT

LAB NUMBER *375*	SAMPLE IDENTIFICATION	ORGANIC MATTER L.O.I. percent	RATE	PHOSPHORUS P1 (WEAK BRAY) 1:7 ppm	RATE	PHOSPHORUS P2 (STRONG BRAY) 1:7 ppm	RATE	PHOSPHORUS OLSEN BICARBONATE P ppm	RATE	POTASSIUM K ppm (NEUTRAL AMMONIUM ACETATE (EXCHANGEABLE))	RATE	MAGNESIUM Mg ppm	RATE	CALCIUM Ca ppm	RATE	SODIUM Na ppm	RATE	pH SOIL pH 1:1	pH BUFFER INDEX	CATION EXCHANGE CAPACITY C.E.C. meq/100g	PERCENT BASE SATURATION (COMPUTED) % K	% Mg	% Ca	% H	% Na
60560	BMLP	9.2	VH	21	M	52	H			42	L	39	L	412	L	15		4.9	5.9	4.6	2.3	7.1	44.8	44.4	1.4
60561	HBNY	4.4	H	11	L	24	M			65	L	115	VH	791	M	10		5.8	6.8	6.3	2.6	15.2	62.8	18.7	0.7

LAB NUMBER *375*	NITRATE-N (FIA) SURFACE ppm	SURFACE lbs/A	SURFACE depth (in)	SUBSOIL 1 ppm	SUBSOIL 1 lbs/A	SUBSOIL 1 depth (in)	SUBSOIL 2 ppm	SUBSOIL 2 lbs/A	SUBSOIL 2 depth (in)	Total lbs/A	SULFUR S ICAP ppm	RATE	ZINC Zn DTPA ppm	RATE	MANGANESE Mn DTPA ppm	RATE	IRON Fe DTPA ppm	RATE	COPPER Cu DTPA ppm	RATE	BORON B SORB. DTPA ppm	RATE	EXCESS LIME RATE	SOLUBLE SALTS 1:1 mmhos/cm	RATE	
60560	22	40	0-6							40	14	M	2.3	M	21	H	95	VH	0.3	VL	0.1	VL	L	0.2	L	
60561	14	25	0-6							25	7	L	0.7	L	16	H	72	VH	0.8	L	0.2	VL	L	0.1	L	

Calcium

20 40.076
Ca
Calcium

Benefits

- Improves soil structure
- Stimulates soil microbes and earthworms
- Mobilizes nutrients into plant
- Increases nitrogen utilization and protein content
- Stimulates root and leaf growth
- Facilitates cell division
- Helps build cell walls
- Improves enzyme function
- Increases sugar content of plant
- Promotes overall plant health
- Produces high-quality grain or fruit

Ideal Levels

- 70–80% of total exchangeable cations
- pH 6.5–7.5

Best Sources

- Eggshells
- Snail or oyster shells
- Animal bones
- (Burning the above three kills any potential human pathogens and converts much of the slowly available calcium carbonate into readily available calcium oxide)
- Limestone kiln dust (LKD)
- Calcium sulfate (gypsum) (23% Ca, 17% S)
- High-calcium lime (low Mg) (30–35% Ca)

Comments

- Calcium is the trucker of all minerals and the key to soil and plant health. Even if the soil test says there is sufficient calcium, adding more soluble calcium, sulfur, and boron is almost always beneficial. If the pH is low, use lime; if it's neutral, use kiln dust, gypsum, or a liquid source. Adding ammonium makes rock phosphate more soluble, and burning lime is the best way to make calcium soluble. When soils are really high in Mg, K, or Na, ideal levels will be hard to achieve and may not be your goal, especially in dry, high CEC soils.

Sodium

"A Dash of Salt"

Sodium is not essential for all plants, but it can be beneficial in many conditions. When potassium is deficient, sodium can fill potassium's role. However, excess sodium can cause problems with water uptake, just like in humans.

SOIL ANALYSIS REPORT

LAB NUMBER *375*	SAMPLE IDENTIFICATION	ORGANIC MATTER L.O.I. percent / RATE	PHOSPHORUS P_1 (WEAK BRAY) 1:7 ppm / RATE	PHOSPHORUS P_2 (STRONG BRAY) 1:7 ppm / RATE	PHOSPHORUS OLSEN BICARBONATE P ppm / RATE	POTASSIUM K ppm / RATE	MAGNESIUM Mg ppm / RATE	CALCIUM Ca ppm / RATE	SODIUM Na ppm / RATE	pH SOIL pH 1:1	pH BUFFER INDEX	CATION EXCHANGE CAPACITY C.E.C. meq/100g	% K	% Mg	% Ca	% H	% Na
60560	BMLP	9.2 VH	21 M	52 H		42 L	39 L	412 L	15	4.9	5.9	4.6	2.3	7.1	44.8	44.4	1.4
60561	HBNY	4.4 H	11 L	24 M		65 L	115 VH	791 M	10	5.8	6.8	6.3	2.6	15.2	62.8	18.7	0.7

(POTASSIUM, MAGNESIUM, CALCIUM, SODIUM: NEUTRAL AMMONIUM ACETATE (EXCHANGEABLE); PERCENT BASE SATURATION (COMPUTED))

LAB NUMBER *375*	NITRATE-N (FIA) SURFACE ppm	SURFACE lbs/A	SURFACE depth (in)	SUBSOIL 1 ppm	SUBSOIL 1 lbs/A	SUBSOIL 1 depth (in)	SUBSOIL 2 ppm	SUBSOIL 2 lbs/A	SUBSOIL 2 depth (in)	Total lbs/A	SULFUR S ICAP ppm / RATE	ZINC Zn DTPA ppm / RATE	MANGANESE Mn DTPA ppm / RATE	IRON Fe DTPA ppm / RATE	COPPER Cu DTPA ppm / RATE	BORON B SORB. DTPA ppm / RATE	EXCESS LIME RATE	SOLUBLE SALTS 1:1 mmhos/cm / RATE	
60560	22	40	0-6							40	14 M	2.3 M	21 H	95 VH	0.3 VL	0.1 VL	L	0.2 L	
60561	14	25	0-6							25	7 L	0.7 L	16 H	72 VH	0.8 L	0.2 VL	L	0.1 L	

Sodium

11 22.990
Na
Sodium

Benefits

- Sodium supports photosynthesis, nutrient transport, and water regulation. It can enhance growth in crops such as sugar beets and celery. It helps suppress phytophthora crown and root rot in crops such as asparagus.

Best Sources

- Numerous OMRI-approved salt products are commercially available and often used as a source of additional trace minerals.

Ideal Levels

- 0.5–3% is considered optimal. Levels exceeding 1% can begin to limit yields. Ideal sodium levels differ by crop.

Comments

- In most soils, excess sodium is more of a problem than deficient sodium. In rare situations, we add Na when it's excessively low. If soil tests high in sodium, it is usually from poor drainage, high-sodium irrigation water, or excessive urea application. Sometimes this can be fixed by adding gypsum and phosphorus. The sodium level should be lower than the P2 phosphorus level on the soil test.
- In grazing operations where the K is really high and cows don't prefer the forages, adding sodium chloride at a few hundred pounds per acre can be beneficial, because Na can replace some K. Soils with sodium levels over 10 percent require different management.

Sulfur

Sulfur is sometimes referred to as the "fourth major nutrient" because it is a key building block in many amino acids, oils, vitamins, and chlorophyll. It is linked to nitrogen consumption through its role in the conversion of nitrate to amino acids.

SOIL ANALYSIS REPORT

LAB NUMBER *375*	SAMPLE IDENTIFICATION	ORGANIC MATTER L.O.I. percent	RATE	PHOSPHORUS P1 (WEAK BRAY) 1:7 ppm	RATE	PHOSPHORUS P2 (STRONG BRAY) 1:7 ppm	RATE	PHOSPHORUS OLSEN BICARBONATE P ppm	RATE	NEUTRAL AMMONIUM ACETATE (EXCHANGEABLE) POTASSIUM K ppm	RATE	MAGNESIUM Mg ppm	RATE	CALCIUM Ca ppm	RATE	SODIUM Na ppm	RATE	pH SOIL pH 1:1	pH BUFFER INDEX	CATION EXCHANGE CAPACITY C.E.C. meq/100g	PERCENT BASE SATURATION (COMPUTED) % K	% Mg	% Ca	% H	% Na
60560	BMLP	9.2	VH	21	M	52	H			42	L	39	L	412	L	15		4.9	5.9	4.6	2.3	7.1	44.8	44.4	1.4
60561	HBNY	4.4	H	11	L	24	M			65	L	115	VH	791	M	10		5.8	6.8	6.3	2.6	15.2	62.8	18.7	0.7

LAB NUMBER *375*	NITRATE-N (FIA) SURFACE ppm	SURFACE lbs/A	SURFACE depth (in)	SUBSOIL 1 ppm	SUBSOIL 1 lbs/A	SUBSOIL 1 depth (in)	SUBSOIL 2 ppm	SUBSOIL 2 lbs/A	SUBSOIL 2 depth (in)	Total lbs/A	SULFUR S ICAP ppm	RATE	ZINC Zn DTPA ppm	RATE	MANGANESE Mn DTPA ppm	RATE	IRON Fe DTPA ppm	RATE	COPPER Cu DTPA ppm	RATE	BORON B SORB. DTPA ppm	RATE	EXCESS LIME RATE	SOLUBLE SALTS 1:1 mmhos/cm	RATE	
60560	22	40	0-6							40	14	M	2.3	M	21	H	95	VH	0.3	VL	0.1	VL	L	0.2	L	
60561	14	25	0-6							25	7	L	0.7	L	16	H	72	VH	0.8	L	0.2	VL	L	0.1	L	

Sulfur

16	32.06
S	
Sulfur	

Benefits

- Essential for synthesis of high-quality, complete protein
- Makes soil nitrogen more available
- Loosens and aerates soil
- Helps reduce excess soil magnesium
- Lowers soil pH
- Facilitates energy release in cells
- Is part of vitamin B and biotin

Best Sources

- Elemental sulfur
- Calcium sulfate (gypsum) (23% Ca, 17% S)
- Potassium sulfate (0-0-50-17S)
- Sulfate trace minerals

Ideal Levels

- Plant N:S ratio of 10–12:1

Comments

- Sulfur helps build humus
- Sulfur helps make deep-green plants
- A plant N:S ratio of 10:1 assures quality proteins and healthy plants. Too much nitrogen can cause pest and disease problems. Elemental sulfur can lower pH and must be converted to a plant-usable form by soil microorganisms. Adding elemental S to compost piles can start to break down and save some N by making ammonium sulfate. If soil S levels get too high, you likely have a drainage problem or a lack of moisture. Anaerobic conditions can be caused by excessive tillage when soil is wet and is detectable by a rotten egg or burned tire smell.

Zinc

A Metabolic Lubricant

Zinc promotes timely, bountiful growth. It is an important component of metabolic enzymes and reactions during plant growth and development. Synthesis of carbohydrates, proteins, and chlorophyll depends on a reliable supply of this critical nutrient.

SOIL ANALYSIS REPORT

LAB NUMBER *375*	SAMPLE IDENTIFICATION	ORGANIC MATTER L.O.I. percent	RATE	PHOSPHORUS P1 (WEAK BRAY) 1:7 ppm	RATE	P2 (STRONG BRAY) 1:7 ppm	RATE	OLSEN - BICARBONATE P ppm	RATE
60560	BMLP	9.2	VH	21	M	52	H		
60561	HBNY	4.4	H	11	L	24	M		

LAB NUMBER *375*	NEUTRAL AMMONIUM ACETATE (EXCHANGEABLE): POTASSIUM K ppm	RATE	MAGNESIUM Mg ppm	RATE	CALCIUM Ca ppm	RATE	SODIUM Na ppm	RATE	pH: SOIL pH 1:1	BUFFER INDEX	CATION EXCHANGE CAPACITY C.E.C. meq/100g	PERCENT BASE SATURATION (COMPUTED): % K	% Mg	% Ca	% H	% Na
60560	42	L	39	L	412	L	15		4.9	5.9	4.6	2.3	7.1	44.8	44.4	1.4
60561	65	L	115	VH	791	M	10		5.8	6.8	6.3	2.6	15.2	62.8	18.7	0.7

LAB NUMBER *375*	NITRATE-N (FIA) SURFACE ppm	lbs/A	depth (in)	SUBSOIL 1 ppm	lbs/A	depth (in)	SUBSOIL 2 ppm	lbs/A	depth (in)	Total lbs/A
60560	22	40	0-6							40
60561	14	25	0-6							25

LAB NUMBER *375*	SULFUR S ICAP ppm	RATE	ZINC Zn DTPA ppm	RATE	MANGANESE Mn DTPA ppm	RATE	IRON Fe DTPA ppm	RATE	COPPER Cu DTPA ppm	RATE	BORON B SORB. DTPA ppm	RATE	EXCESS LIME RATE	SOLUBLE SALTS 1:1 mmhos/cm	RATE	
60560	14	M	2.3	M	21	H	95	VH	0.3	VL	0.1	VL	L	0.2	L	
60561	7	L	0.7	L	16	H	72	VH	0.8	L	0.2	VL	L	0.1	L	

Zinc

30 65.38
Zn
Zinc

Benefits

- Contributes to test weight
- Increases ear size in maize
- Promotes silking in maize
- Hastens maturity
- Promotes chlorophyll formation
- Improves enzyme function
- Regulates plant growth
- Increases plant leaf size

Best Sources

- Zinc sulfate (35% Zn)

Ideal Levels

- 5–10 ppm on soil test. Higher levels in high-P soils.
- P:Zn ratio of 10:1 is optimal but not always achievable.

Comments

- Extremely important in phosphorus uptake and utilization within the plant.
- Zinc deficiency appears to be a common micronutrient deficiency in crop plants. It is particularly common in high-pH soils.

Manganese

Manganese helps plants "breathe." Plants only need Mn in small quantities, but it is critical to growth. It aids in the collection and release of energy during photosynthesis and is also important for the nitrogen cycle within the plant.

SOIL ANALYSIS REPORT

LAB NUMBER *375*	SAMPLE IDENTIFICATION	ORGANIC MATTER L.O.I. percent	RATE	PHOSPHORUS P1 (WEAK BRAY) 1:7 ppm	RATE	PHOSPHORUS P2 (STRONG BRAY) 1:7 ppm	RATE	PHOSPHORUS OLSEN BICARBONATE P ppm	RATE	NEUTRAL AMMONIUM ACETATE (EXCHANGEABLE): POTASSIUM K ppm	RATE	MAGNESIUM Mg ppm	RATE	CALCIUM Ca ppm	RATE	SODIUM Na ppm	RATE	pH: SOIL pH 1:1	BUFFER INDEX	CATION EXCHANGE CAPACITY C.E.C. meq/100g	PERCENT BASE SATURATION (COMPUTED): % K	% Mg	% Ca	% H	% Na
60560	BMLP	9.2	VH	21	M	52	H			42	L	39	L	412	L	15		4.9	5.9	4.6	2.3	7.1	44.8	44.4	1.4
60561	HBNY	4.4	H	11	L	24	M			65	L	115	VH	791	M	10		5.8	6.8	6.3	2.6	15.2	62.8	18.7	0.7

LAB NUMBER *375*	NITRATE-N (FIA): SURFACE ppm	SURFACE lbs/A	SURFACE depth (in)	SUBSOIL 1 ppm	SUBSOIL 1 lbs/A	SUBSOIL 1 depth (in)	SUBSOIL 2 ppm	SUBSOIL 2 lbs/A	SUBSOIL 2 depth (in)	Total lbs/A	SULFUR S ICAP ppm	RATE	ZINC Zn DTPA ppm	RATE	MANGANESE Mn DTPA ppm	RATE	IRON Fe DTPA ppm	RATE	COPPER Cu DTPA ppm	RATE	BORON B SORB. DTPA ppm	RATE	EXCESS LIME RATE	SOLUBLE SALTS 1:1 mmhos/cm	RATE	
60560	22	40	0-6							40	14	M	2.3	M	21	H	95	VH	0.3	VL	0.1	VL	L	0.2	L	
60561	14	25	0-6							25	7	L	0.7	L	16	H	72	VH	0.8	L	0.2	VL	L	0.1	L	

Manganese

25 54.938
Mn
Manganese

Benefits

- Normal growth and photosynthesis
- Oil production
- Energy release in cells
- Enzyme functions

Best Sources

- Manganese sulfate

Ideal Levels

- Fe:Mn ratio of 1:2

Comments

- Involved in nitrogen mobility and utilization within the plant.
- Because manganese is a biological mineral, levels in the plant can be high even if soil test results show low levels. Soil test results can vary widely depending on the extraction method used by the lab. Before buying lots of Mn, you do need to measure plant uptake. If plant tissue levels are high in both P and Mn, soil biology must be working. Some specialty crops like blueberries require a lot of manganese, which is more likely to get into the plant at low pH levels.

Iron

Iron is the most common metallic element on the planet and is important for plant health. It is critical for chlorophyll synthesis and is an essential micronutrient for plant development. Soil pH determines the availability of iron and other micronutrients to plants.

SOIL ANALYSIS REPORT

LAB NUMBER *375*	SAMPLE IDENTIFICATION	ORGANIC MATTER L.O.I. percent	RATE	PHOSPHORUS P1 (WEAK BRAY) 1:7 ppm	RATE	PHOSPHORUS P2 (STRONG BRAY) 1:7 ppm	RATE	PHOSPHORUS OLSEN BICARBONATE P ppm	RATE	NEUTRAL AMMONIUM ACETATE (EXCHANGEABLE) POTASSIUM K ppm	RATE	MAGNESIUM Mg ppm	RATE	CALCIUM Ca ppm	RATE	SODIUM Na ppm	RATE	pH SOIL pH 1:1	pH BUFFER INDEX	CATION EXCHANGE CAPACITY C.E.C. meq/100g	PERCENT BASE SATURATION (COMPUTED) % K	% Mg	% Ca	% H	% Na
60560	BMLP	9.2	VH	21	M	52	H			42	L	39	L	412	L	15		4.9	5.9	4.6	2.3	7.1	44.8	44.4	1.4
60561	HBNY	4.4	H	11	L	24	M			65	L	115	VH	791	M	10		5.8	6.8	6.3	2.6	15.2	62.8	18.7	0.7

LAB NUMBER *375*	NITRATE-N (FIA) SURFACE ppm	SURFACE lbs/A	SURFACE depth (in)	SUBSOIL 1 ppm	SUBSOIL 1 lbs/A	SUBSOIL 1 depth (in)	SUBSOIL 2 ppm	SUBSOIL 2 lbs/A	SUBSOIL 2 depth (in)	Total lbs/A	SULFUR S ICAP ppm	RATE	ZINC Zn DTPA ppm	RATE	MANGANESE Mn DTPA ppm	RATE	IRON Fe DTPA ppm	RATE	COPPER Cu DTPA ppm	RATE	BORON B SORB. DTPA ppm	RATE	EXCESS LIME RATE	SOLUBLE SALTS 1:1 mmhos/cm	RATE	
60560	22	40	0-6							40	14	M	2.3	M	21	H	95	VH	0.3	VL	0.1	VL	L	0.2	L	
60561	14	25	0-6							25	7	L	0.7	L	16	H	72	VH	0.8	L	0.2	VL	L	0.1	L	

Iron

26 55.845
Fe
Iron

Benefits

- Chlorophyll production
- Energy release in cells
- Needed by nitrogen-fixing bacteria

Best Sources

- Iron sulfate

Ideal Levels

- 20 ppm or 40 pounds per acre

Comments

- High iron ties up phosphorus
- Watch for excessive iron in animal feed, especially for horses and swine
- High iron in the soil makes phosphorus less available
- Iron is strongly influenced by pH, and excess is often a bigger problem than deficiency. Excess iron uptake can be slowed by liming.

Copper

Copper helps form lignin in cell walls, which provide support for plants. It is particularly important in the formation of viable pollen, seed set, and stress resistance. It is also required for enzymatic activities, as well as chlorophyll and seed production.

SOIL ANALYSIS REPORT

LAB NUMBER *375*	SAMPLE IDENTIFICATION	ORGANIC MATTER L.O.I. percent	ORGANIC MATTER RATE	PHOSPHORUS P_1 (WEAK BRAY) 1:7 ppm	P_1 RATE	PHOSPHORUS P_2 (STRONG BRAY) 1:7 ppm	P_2 RATE	PHOSPHORUS OLSEN BICARBONATE P ppm	OLSEN RATE	NEUTRAL AMMONIUM ACETATE (EXCHANGEABLE) POTASSIUM K ppm	K RATE	MAGNESIUM Mg ppm	Mg RATE	CALCIUM Ca ppm	Ca RATE	SODIUM Na ppm	Na RATE	pH SOIL pH 1:1	pH BUFFER INDEX	CATION EXCHANGE CAPACITY C.E.C. meq/100g	PERCENT BASE SATURATION (COMPUTED) % K	% Mg	% Ca	% H	% Na
60560	BMLP	9.2	VH	21	M	52	H			42	L	39	L	412	L	15		4.9	5.9	4.6	2.3	7.1	44.8	44.4	1.4
60561	HBNY	4.4	H	11	L	24	M			65	L	115	VH	791	M	10		5.8	6.8	6.3	2.6	15.2	62.8	18.7	0.7

LAB NUMBER *375*	NITRATE-N (FIA) SURFACE ppm	SURFACE lbs/A	SURFACE depth (in)	SUBSOIL 1 ppm	SUBSOIL 1 lbs/A	SUBSOIL 1 depth (in)	SUBSOIL 2 ppm	SUBSOIL 2 lbs/A	SUBSOIL 2 depth (in)	Total lbs/A	SULFUR S ICAP ppm	S RATE	ZINC Zn DTPA ppm	Zn RATE	MANGANESE Mn DTPA ppm	Mn RATE	IRON Fe DTPA ppm	Fe RATE	COPPER Cu DTPA ppm	Cu RATE	BORON B SORB. DTPA ppm	B RATE	EXCESS LIME RATE	SOLUBLE SALTS 1:1 mmhos/cm	SOLUBLE SALTS RATE
60560	22	40	0-6							40	14	M	2.3	M	21	H	95	VH	**0.3**	**VL**	0.1	VL	L	0.2	L
60561	14	25	0-6							25	7	L	0.7	L	16	H	72	VH	**0.8**	**L**	0.2	VL	L	0.1	L

Copper

29 63.546
Cu
Copper

Benefits

- Helps control mold and fungi
- Benefits photosynthesis
- Releases energy in cells
- Improves enzyme function
- Enhances normal leaf growth
- Increases stalk strength

Best Sources

- Copper sulfate (25% Cu)

Ideal Levels

- 2–5 ppm in soil test. Up to 10 ppm appears to be okay.

Comments

- Involved with the immune systems of plants.
- Helps produce high-quality crops with greater storability.
- Copper has many benefits for plant and soil function, such as controlling fungal diseases. Because copper sulfate is a fungicide, fall application for soil correction is best.

Boron

Boron plays a major role in the function of cell walls and influences many parts of the plant, including roots, stem cells, pollen, and seeds. Boron assists in the uptake of calcium and the function of several metabolic pathways, most notably translocation of sugars within the plant.

SOIL ANALYSIS REPORT

LAB NUMBER *375*	SAMPLE IDENTIFICATION	ORGANIC MATTER L.O.I. percent	ORGANIC MATTER RATE	PHOSPHORUS P1 (WEAK BRAY) 1:7 ppm	RATE	PHOSPHORUS P2 (STRONG BRAY) 1:7 ppm	RATE	OLSEN BICARBONATE P ppm	RATE	POTASSIUM K ppm	RATE	MAGNESIUM Mg ppm	RATE	CALCIUM Ca ppm	RATE	SODIUM Na ppm	RATE	pH SOIL pH 1:1	pH BUFFER INDEX	CATION EXCHANGE CAPACITY C.E.C. meq/100g	PERCENT BASE SATURATION (COMPUTED) % K	% Mg	% Ca	% H	% Na
60560	BMLP	9.2	VH	21	M	52	H			42	L	39	L	412	L	15		4.9	5.9	4.6	2.3	7.1	44.8	44.4	1.4
60561	HBNY	4.4	H	11	L	24	M			65	L	115	VH	791	M	10		5.8	6.8	6.3	2.6	15.2	62.8	18.7	0.7

(Potassium, magnesium, calcium and sodium: NEUTRAL AMMONIUM ACETATE (EXCHANGEABLE))

LAB NUMBER *375*	NITRATE-N (FIA) SURFACE ppm	SURFACE lbs/A	SURFACE depth (in)	SUBSOIL 1 ppm	SUBSOIL 1 lbs/A	SUBSOIL 1 depth (in)	SUBSOIL 2 ppm	SUBSOIL 2 lbs/A	SUBSOIL 2 depth (in)	Total lbs/A	SULFUR S ICAP ppm	RATE	ZINC Zn DTPA ppm	RATE	MANGANESE Mn DTPA ppm	RATE	IRON Fe DTPA ppm	RATE	COPPER Cu DTPA ppm	RATE	**BORON B SORB. DTPA ppm**	**RATE**	EXCESS LIME RATE	SOLUBLE SALTS 1:1 mmhos/cm	RATE
60560	22	40	0-6							40	14	M	2.3	M	21	H	95	VH	0.3	VL	**0.1**	**VL**	L	0.2	L
60561	14	25	0-6							25	7	L	0.7	L	16	H	72	VH	0.8	L	**0.2**	**VL**	L	0.1	L

Boron

5 10.81
B
Boron

Benefits

- Promotes flowering and pollen (silk and tassel in maize)
- Seed development
- Root and leaf growth
- Cell wall formation
- Protein production
- Sugar translocation
- Energy release in cells
- Improves quality
- Increases calcium uptake

Best Sources

- Calcium borate (14% B)
- Sodium borate (Borax. Yes, the laundry detergent booster.)
- Soil organic matter

Ideal Levels

- 2 ppm in soil test is ideal but rarely achieved

Comments

- The "gate opener" to put calcium in the plant.
- Don't expect mineral uptake without addressing boron.
- Needs to be addressed yearly because it is so highly water-soluble.
- Do not use sodium borate on salty soils.
- Balancing soil levels of boron, an anion, are difficult because it leaches just like N and S. Providing some in the crop fertilizer is needed on most farms. Adding boron to nitrogen and calcium sources is a good idea. Boron is the most limiting trace element on most farms.

Nitrogen

Amino Acids, Proteins, and More!

Nitrogen is the only element that can be grown on the farm, where symbiotic soil bacteria fix it from the atmosphere. Legumes, soil bacteria, plant symbiotic relations, and young, highly digestible plants provide N. Nitrogen is a necessary evil. Don't provide more than is absolutely needed. Splitting applications or adding carbon with the N are good ideas. Excessive nitrogen can have a negative effect on plant and soil health. Aim for a good carbon:nitrogen ratio.

SOIL ANALYSIS REPORT

LAB NUMBER *375*	SAMPLE IDENTIFICATION	ORGANIC MATTER L.O.I. percent	ORGANIC MATTER RATE	PHOSPHORUS P (WEAK BRAY) 1:7 ppm	RATE	PHOSPHORUS P_2 (STRONG BRAY) 1:7 ppm	RATE	PHOSPHORUS OLSEN BICARBONATE P ppm	RATE	NEUTRAL AMMONIUM ACETATE (EXCHANGEABLE) POTASSIUM K ppm	RATE	MAGNESIUM Mg ppm	RATE	CALCIUM Ca ppm	RATE	SODIUM Na ppm	RATE	pH SOIL pH 1:1	pH BUFFER INDEX	CATION EXCHANGE CAPACITY C.E.C. meq/100g	PERCENT BASE SATURATION (COMPUTED) % K	% Mg	% Ca	% H	% Na
60560	BMLP	9.2	VH	21	M	52	H			42	L	39	L	412	L	15		4.9	5.9	4.6	2.3	7.1	44.8	44.4	1.4
60561	HBNY	4.4	H	11	L	24	M			65	L	115	VH	791	M	10		5.8	6.8	6.3	2.6	15.2	62.8	18.7	0.7

LAB NUMBER *375*	NITRATE-N (FIA) SURFACE ppm	SURFACE lbs/A	SURFACE depth (in)	SUBSOIL 1 ppm	SUBSOIL 1 lbs/A	SUBSOIL 1 depth (in)	SUBSOIL 2 ppm	SUBSOIL 2 lbs/A	SUBSOIL 2 depth (in)	Total lbs/A	SULFUR S ICAP ppm	RATE	ZINC Zn DTPA ppm	RATE	MANGANESE Mn DTPA ppm	RATE	IRON Fe DTPA ppm	RATE	COPPER Cu DTPA ppm	RATE	BORON B SORB. DTPA ppm	RATE	EXCESS LIME RATE	SOLUBLE SALTS 1:1 mmhos/cm	RATE
60560	22	40	0-6							40	14	M	2.3	M	21	H	95	VH	0.3	VL	0.1	VL	L	0.2	L
60561	14	25	0-6							25	7	L	0.7	L	16	H	72	VH	0.8	L	0.2	VL	L	0.1	L

Nitrogen

7 14.007

N

Nitrogen

Benefits

- The driver of chlorophyll production
- Benefits photosynthesis
- Stimulates vigorous, leafy growth
- A key component of DNA, amino acids, and proteins

Best Sources

- Livestock manure, legume and other green manure crops, fish products, compost, alfalfa meal, soybean meal, feather meal
- Healthy, mineral-balanced soils with adequate organic matter and an active soil life

Ideal Levels

- 25 ppm to 30 ppm is considered the "critical threshold" for optimal growth. Amounts beyond this may not utilized and can lead to nitrate leaching

Comments

- Splitting applications of N or adding carbon with it provide adequate levels without short-term excess
- Excess N "burns" off soil carbon, can have negative effects on plant growth and forage quality, and can cause insect issues and fungal diseases
- Ammonium sulfate provides sulfur as well as nitrogen

Keys to Quality Forages

With good mineral balance, proper fertility, and healthy soils, the feed or food quality changes. Feeds have increased energy, higher digestibility, and more digestible fibers. A good balance will also increase feed mineral content, and adequate balancing and sulfur levels will improve protein quality. Livestock fed forages grown on properly balanced soil will perform better and be healthier on a diet with a higher percent of forage.

As a dairy nutritionist, I have tested a lot of forages. Animals perform best when the big four nutrients are high in the plant—calcium, phosphorus, magnesium, and boron.

Calcium rarely gets in plants by just having the correct pH. Soluble sources need to be added along with *boron*. *Phosphorus* is a biological mineral and may not be plant-available even at high soil numbers. It is a great indicator of biological activity. *Magnesium* requires managed potassium levels, additives, and the use of sulfur to form magnesium sulfate for plant uptake.

The forage also needs to be digested and have a 10:1 N:S ratio for quality forage performance and to have all the minerals balanced.

Homegrown Nutrients

Nutrients are often available in natural waste products. Making efficient use of these products can increase resiliency and decrease costs.

Manure is more than a waste product. It can supply valuable nutrients for crop production, including **nitrogen**, **potassium**, **phosphorus**, and **organic matter**. Its value depends on the type of livestock, the diet fed, bedding type, physical characteristics (solid, semi-solid, or liquid), proper storage, and application.

Compost is decomposed manure and includes the same nutrient benefits as manure, but nutrients are more stable and soil-friendly.

The availability and nutrient quality of manure and compost is figured into recommendations. Farms with adequate manure may only need to add calcium, sulfur, and micronutrients.

Green manure crops may be used to provide nutrients, including nitrogen for the crop and food microbes. Oats, buckwheat, rye, ryegrass, and hairy vetch are some examples of common green manure crops.

Plowing down alfalfa can provide significant amounts of nitrogen and other benefits.

Use of these natural nutrient production methods may significantly decrease the need to purchase fertilizers.

Compost teas: Although compost tea will contain some levels of fertilizer nutrients, it is primarily a "starter solution" full of microorganisms. When applied to the soil, these organisms decompose soil organic matter, releasing the nutrients held inside. Compost teas can be aerated or non-aerated. Molasses can be added in order to rapidly multiply microorganism populations. It should be used quickly, while organisms are still active and alive.

Fermented Plant Juice (FPJ): Green plants fermented in water contain highly available plant nutrients. FPJ from legumes generally contains more nitrogen. Ferments of unripe fruits are high in phosphorus, and plants such as comfrey and dandelion greens are high in potassium. FPJ delivers enzymes, hormones, and microbes.

Ramial chipped wood (RCW): Young tree and shrub branches contain most of the plant's mineral nutrients. Chipped small-diameter wood can be applied as a mulch, lightly incorporated into the soil, steeped like compost tea, or fermented. Agroforestry systems, especially using nitrogen-fixing trees that can be cut-and-come-again, can produce most of a farm's fertilizer needs.

Basic Principles

1. Good decisions can only be made based on complete and accurate information. We want farmers to have the knowledge to analyze information, ask better questions, and make better decisions. We start with a complete soil test that not only measures N-P-K, but also includes other nutrients that plants require for growth. We then recommend a complete program, not just individual products.
2. Soil tests do not measure the total minerals of the soil; they measure minerals that are easily available to the plant. With improved plant root systems, soil aeration, and soil biology, more nutrients can be made available for plant use from soil reserves.
3. A soil teeming with microbial life and earthworms provides additional feed to the crop for growth and performance. Soil life needs to have an ideal home, be protected, and be fed.
4. There is more to a soil fertility program than N-P-K. There are many other nutrients vital to plant growth, including calcium, magnesium, sulfur, zinc, manganese, iron, copper, and boron.
5. Sulfur, boron, and nitrogen are important elements which need to be addressed every year because they are anions and therefore highly leachable.
6. Even if soil pH is in an acceptable range, available calcium may still be low.
7. The productivity of soil can never be greater than the plant food element in least supply. If your soil has enough P and K, where is the economic return of adding more? Why not address calcium and sulfur, which starts the process of soil balancing?
8. The amount of nutrients removed varies with the crop and the crop quality. For example, average alfalfa with 1.2% calcium removes 24 pounds of calcium per acre per ton of yield. At 1.6% calcium, alfalfa removes 32 pounds of calcium per acre per ton of yield.
9. Many times, farmers are able to grow most of their needed nutrients. High biomass-producing agroforestry systems generate a surplus of compostable organic matter while fixing atmospheric nitrogen in the soil. Using nitrogen-fixing woody species such as Black Alder (*Alnus glutinosa*), Black Locust (*Robinia pseudoacacia*) and Eastern Redbud (*Cercis canadensis*) in temperate zones and acacia species such as Faidherbia and Gliricidia in the subtropics to tropics within alley cropping systems can supply all of a crop's N-P-K needs.
10. One of the main reasons for testing soils on livestock farms is to ensure proper utilization of manure and to maintain proper mineral balance.
11. Recommendations may include more than fertilizer products. Other factors affecting soil health such as crop rotations, soil tilth, soil structure, and tillage practices will be evaluated.
12. Nutrient requirements on organic farms are the same as all other farms. The sources of nutrients will vary and need to meet organic farming regulations.

Conclusions

Our approach to soil balancing is to raise the levels of low or deficient elements and to lower (or at least not raise) excess element levels. Since we are dealing mostly with mineral products, this will take several years. It may not be possible to balance some soils to "ideal" proportions, but moving them closer to the ideal will still improve crop performance. When you balance minerals, optimize appropriate tillage, optimize living plant cover, and incorporate livestock into your farming or ranching system, yields will increase in volume and quality, weed pressure will decline, and pests and diseases will no longer present the catastrophic threat that they once did.

Your individual context may necessitate that your efforts be concentrated on "in-row support" in the early years. Mineral amendments can be applied at planting or band-applied later in the season, or perhaps a well-balanced crop fertilizer can be used. You don't necessarily need to correct all of the soil at once. We strive for progress, not perfection, which is the most economical and practical method.

Soil testing, balancing, and supplying the minerals is the project. The feed test or tissue test is the report card. You do need to monitor to see if your program is working.

Other Titles from Acres U.S.A. Books:

Restoration Agriculture
By Mark Shepard

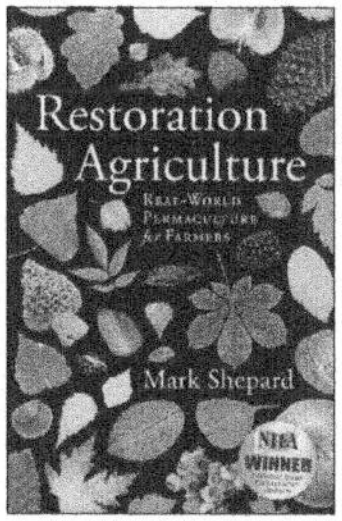

Around the globe, most people get their calories from "annual" agriculture—plants that grow fast for one season, produce lots of seeds, then die. Every single human society that has relied on annual crops for staple foods has collapsed. *Restoration Agriculture* explains how we can have all of the benefits of natural, perennial ecosystems and create agricultural systems that imitate nature in form and function while still providing for our food, building, fuel and many other needs—in your own backyard, farm, or ranch. Based on real-world practices, this book presents an alternative to the agriculture system of eradication and offers exciting hope for our future.

The Biological Farmer
By Gary Zimmer

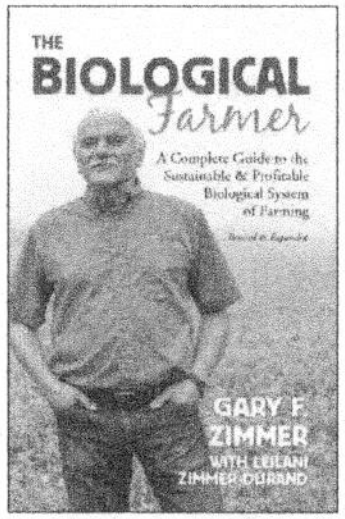

Biological farmers work with nature, feeding soil life, balancing soil minerals, and tilling soils with a purpose. The methods they apply involve a unique system of beliefs, observations and guidelines that result in increased production and profit. This practical how-to guide explains their methods and will help you make farming profitable and fun. Biological farming does not mean less production; it means eliminating obstacles to healthy, efficient production. Once the chemical, physical, and biological properties of the soil are in balance, you can expect optimal outputs, even in bad years. Biological farming improves the environment, reduces erosion, reduces disease and insect problems, and alters weed pressure—and it accomplishes this by working in harmony with nature.

A Growers Guide for Balancing Soils
By William McKibben

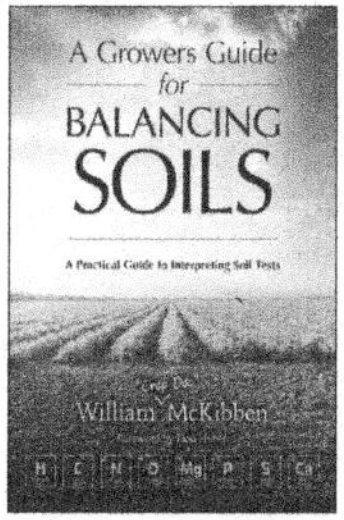

Whether you're a serious home gardener or a full-time farmer, A Growers Guide for Balancing Soils will help you expand your understanding of the science behind plant nutrition. It all starts with the soil, but, as you'll read, just spreading compost and hoping for the best isn't a strategy for success.

Drawing on 40 years of experience using the Albrecht philosophy of balancing soils, William McKibben will walk you through a data-driven, time-tested process that starts with soil analysis, but doesn't stop there. Productive soil that has the right balance of bio-available minerals and maximizes crop production and quality is the goal, and McKibben outlines a common-sense approach for how to get there.